Yes, Yes, Yes! I Matter Too!

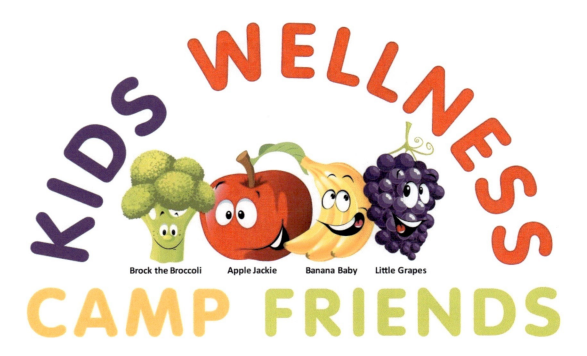

KIDS WELLNESS

Brock the Broccoli   Apple Jackie   Banana Baby   Little Grapes

CAMP FRIENDS

Josie Christine

AuthorHouse™
1663 Liberty Drive
Bloomington, IN 47403
www.authorhouse.com
Phone: 1 (800) 839-8640

Because of the dynamic nature of the Internet, any web addresses or links contained in this book may have changed
since publication and may no longer be valid. The views expressed in this work are solely those of the author and do
not necessarily reflect the views of the publisher, and the publisher hereby disclaims any responsibility for them.

Any people depicted in stock imagery provided by Getty Images are models,
and such images are being used for illustrative purposes only.
Certain stock imagery © Getty Images.

This book is printed on acid-free paper.

ISBN: 978-1-7283-3786-9 (sc)
ISBN: 978-1-7283-3788-3 (hc)
ISBN: 978-1-7283-3787-6 (e)

Library of Congress Control Number: 2019919377

Print information available on the last page.

Published by AuthorHouse 12/21/2019

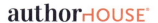

Yes, Yes, Yes!
I Matter Too!

Kids Wellness Camp Friends

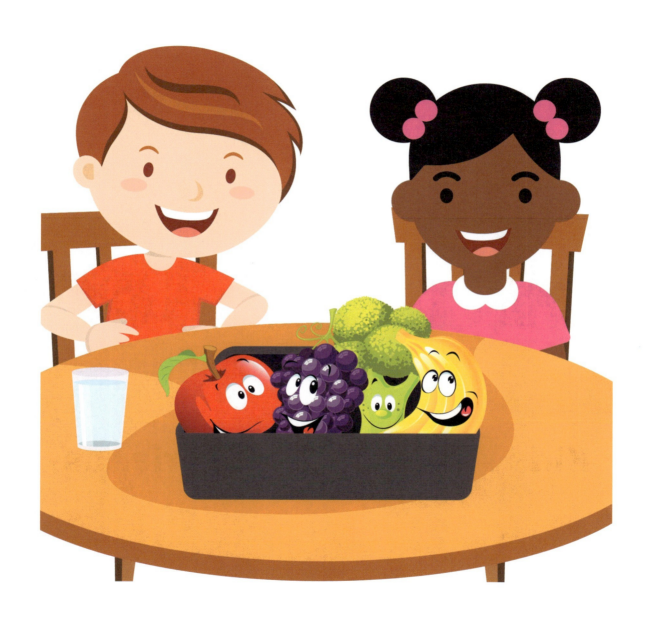

Yes, Yes, Yes! I Matter Too

Yes, Yes, Yes! Oh Yes, I Do!

Shouts four friends all neat in a bunch

Freshly washed and ready for lunch.

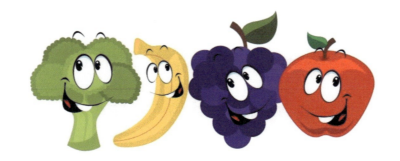

Brock the Broccoli, Apple Jackie,
Banana Baby, and Little Grapes

Sit together and happily wait

Each has a benefit that will last and last

Fruits and veggies the star of the class

Apples, bananas, and grapes are fruits

Each helps you grow big and smile so cute

Look at your skin beautiful and bright

Less coughs and sniffles at night

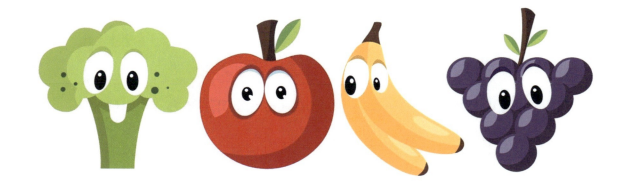

Brock has a sad face toward the other three

Oh well what benefits come from me

I am a vegetable; do I matter too?

Yes, Yes, Yes! Oh, yes, you do!

Broccoli is a veggie that packs a big punch

of tasty goodness with each crunch

Vegetables are fun to eat just like fruit

Yes, Yes, Yes! You do matter too!

Brock is so green, healthy and well

Apple Jackie is crisp and doing quite swell

No more will her friend say what do I do

Yes, Yes, Yes! You do matter too!

Banana Baby is ripe and full of appeal

Good for the heart and helping bones heal

No more will its friend say what do I do

Yes, Yes, Yes! You do matter too!

Little Grapes all packed nice and tight

Building skin cells to fight nasty nights

Wow you are my friend, and I am proud of you

Yes, Yes, Yes! You do matter too!

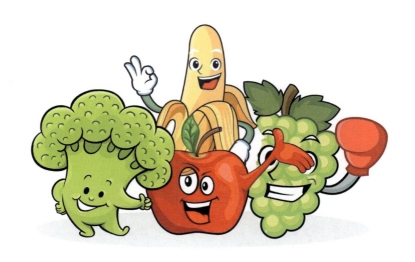

Full of giggles the four friends unite

Now knowing they all matter with every bite

Each packed up for lunch and ready for school

Shouting

Yes, Yes, Yes! We do matter too!

Food with Benefit Alphabet

From A-Z

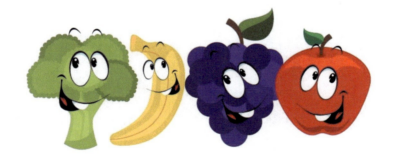

A

ASPARAGUS

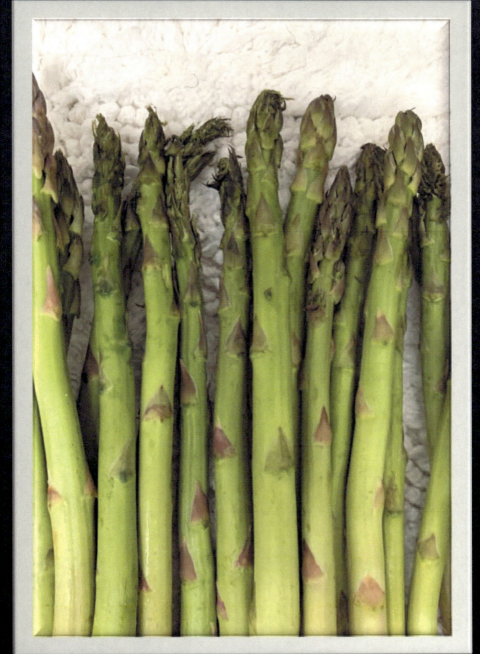

B

BANANA

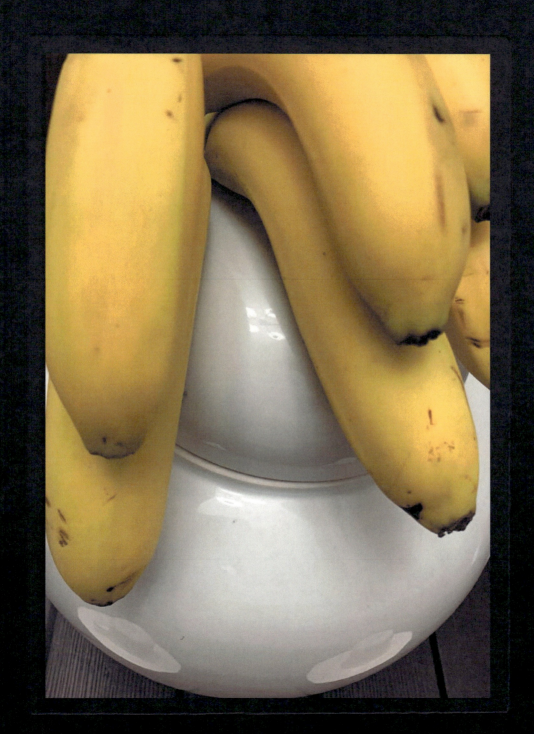

C

CARROT

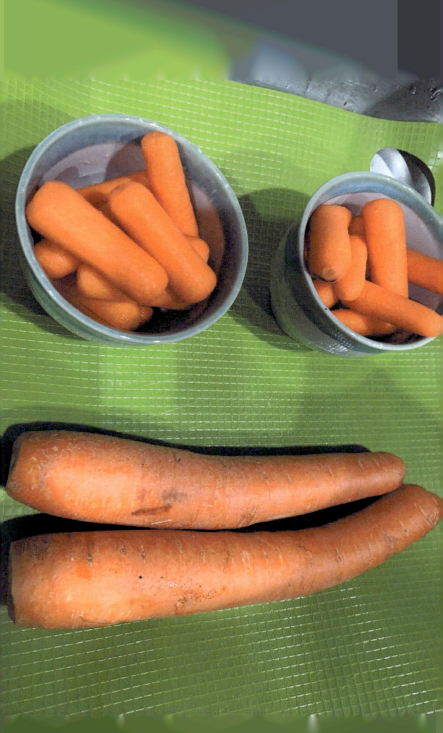

D

DILL

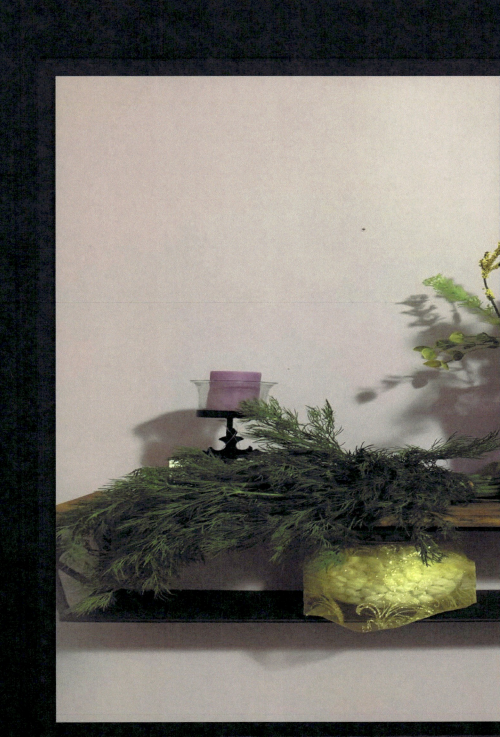

E
EGGPLANT

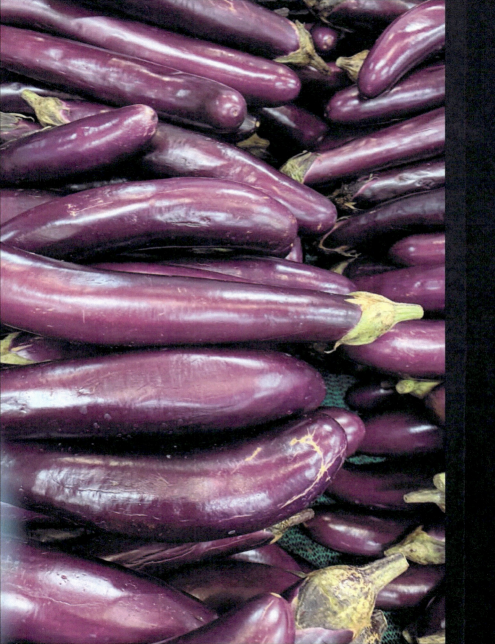

F

FIG

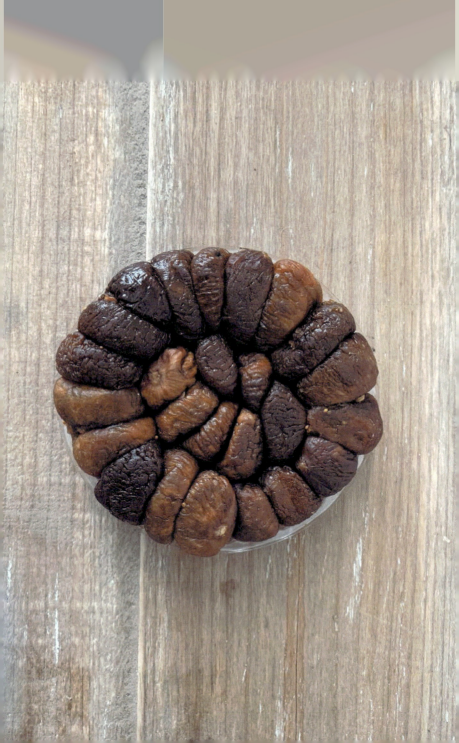

G

GRAPES

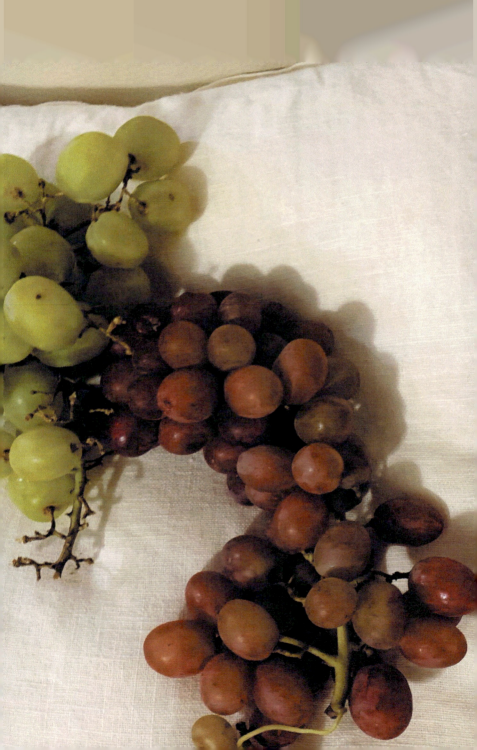

H

HONEYDEW

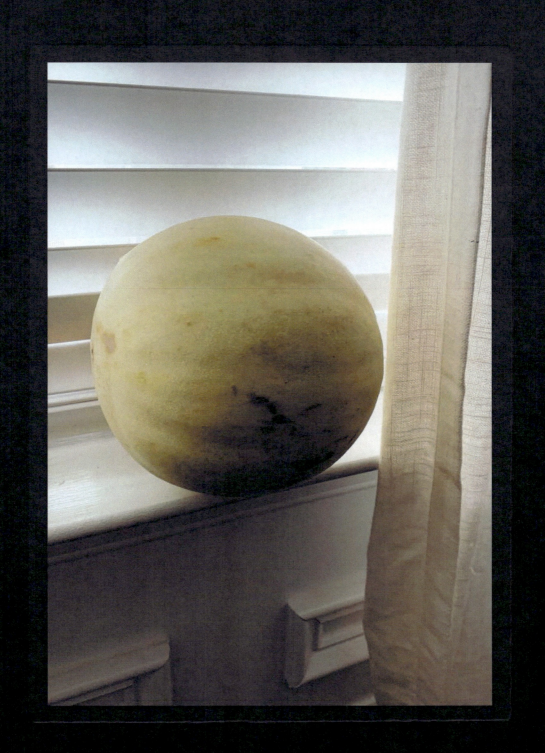

I
ICEBERG
LETTUCE

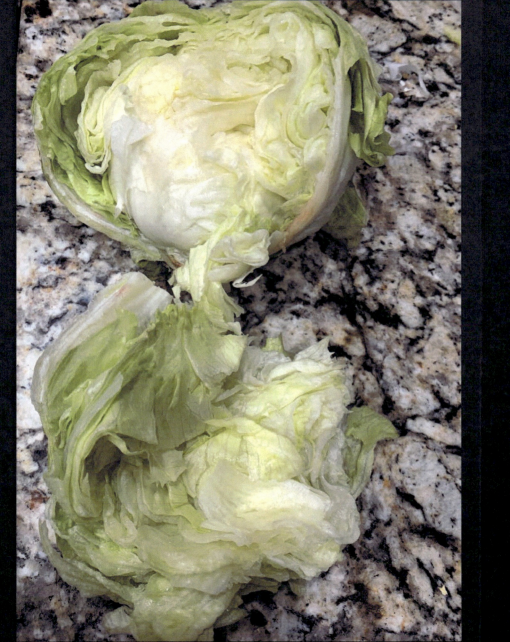

J

JALAPENO

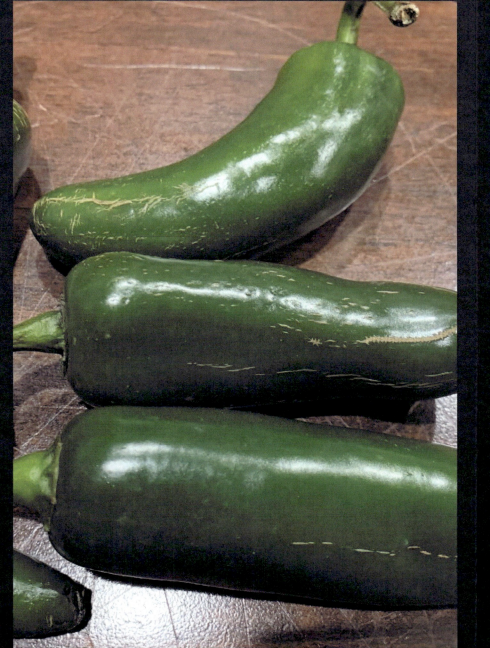

K

KALE

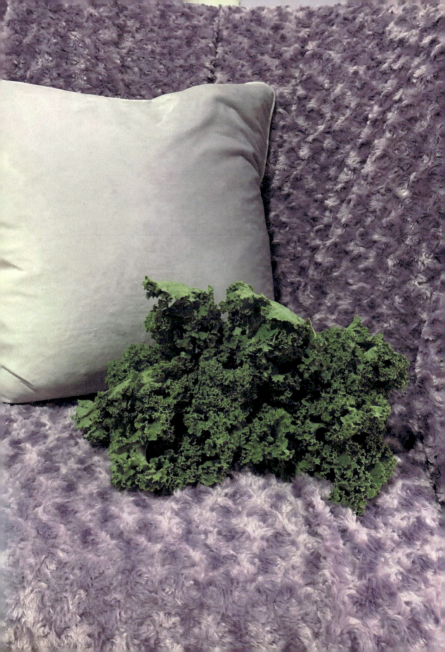

L
LEEKS

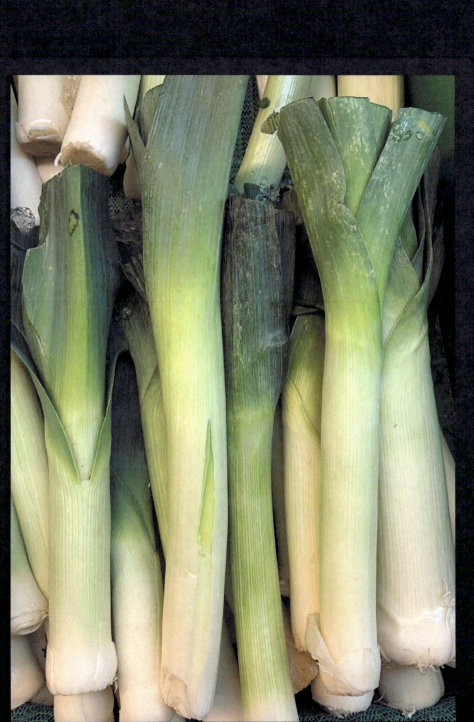

M

MANGO

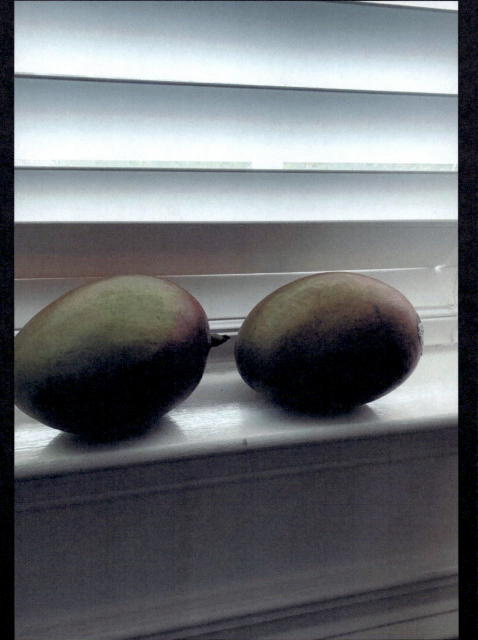

N

NAPA
CABBAGE

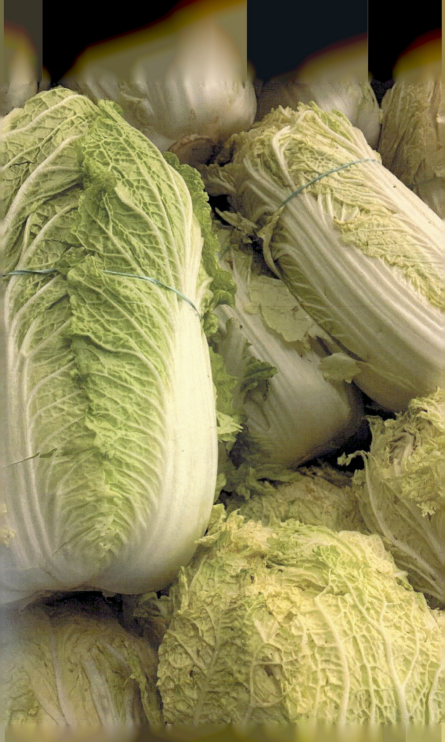

O

ORANGES

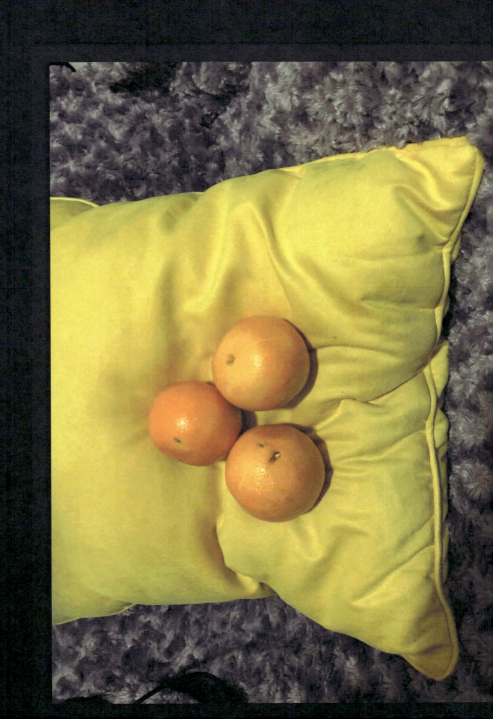

P

PEAS

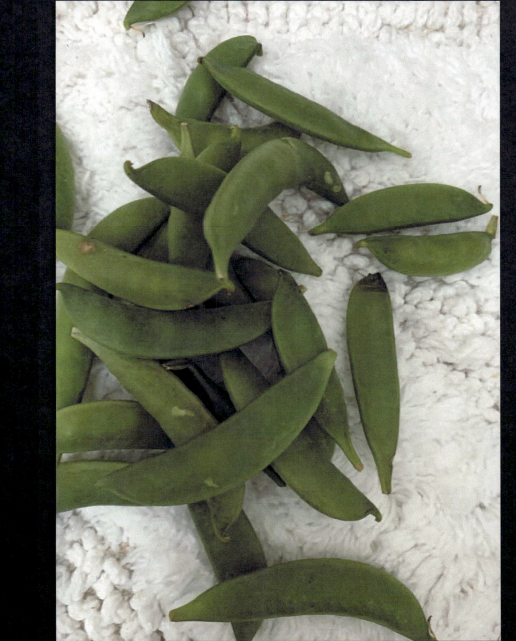

Q

QUINOA

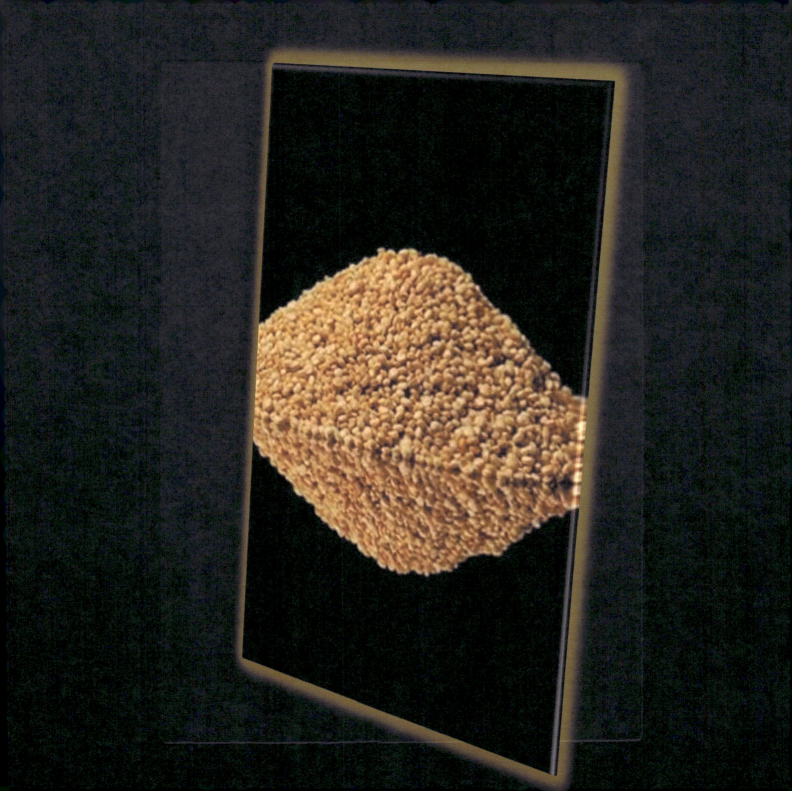

R

RUTABAGA

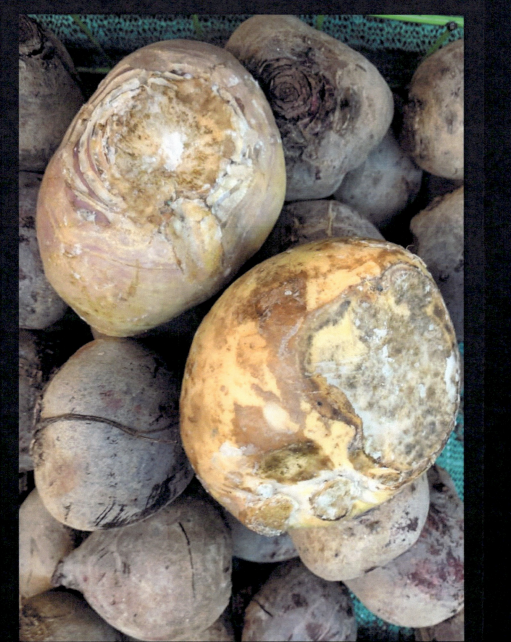

S

SPINACH

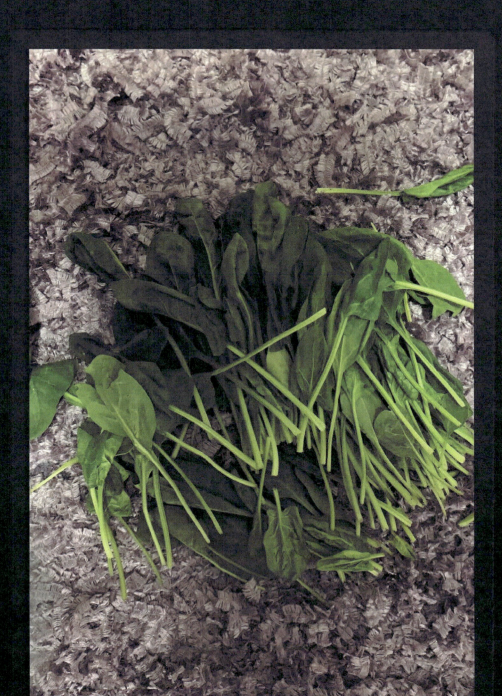

T

TOMATO

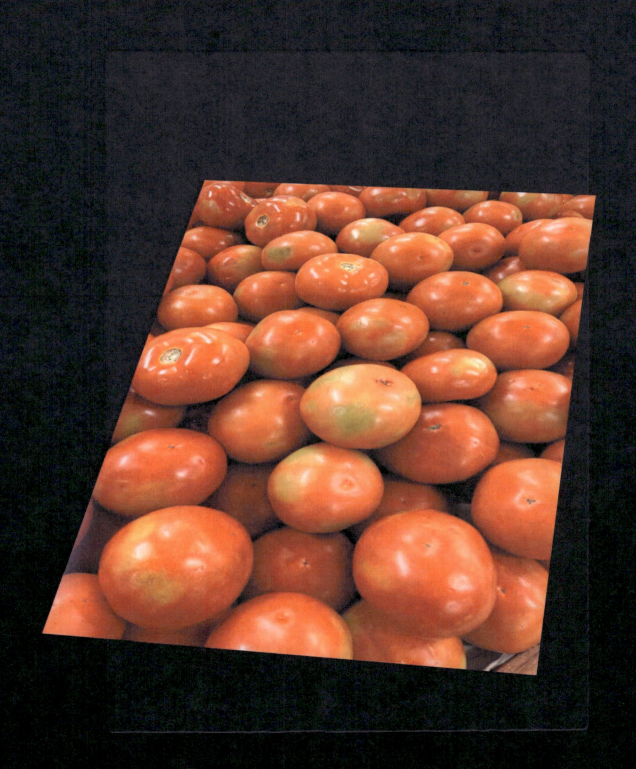

U

UGLI

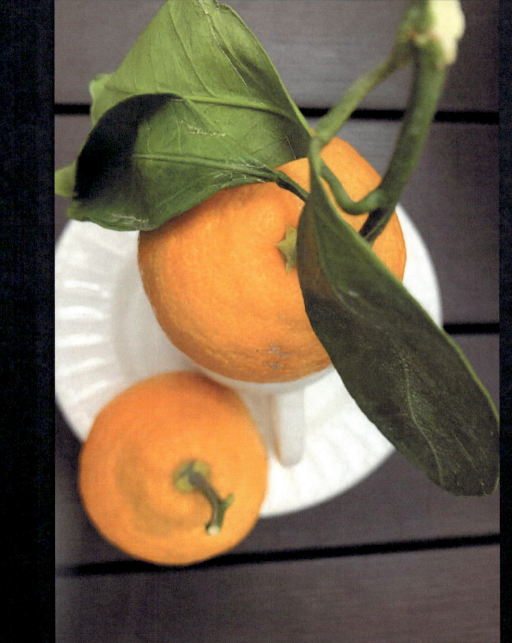

V

VANILLA

Bean

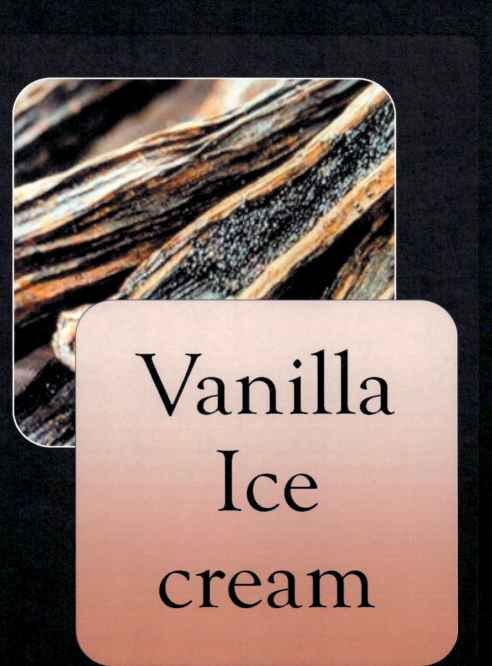

Vanilla
Ice
cream

WATERMELON

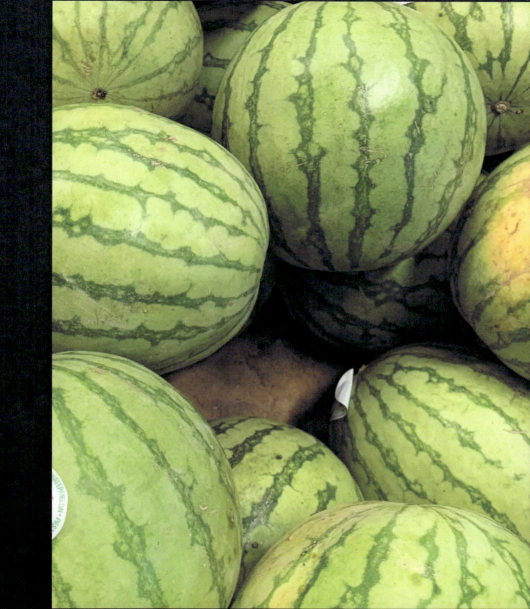

X

XIMENIA

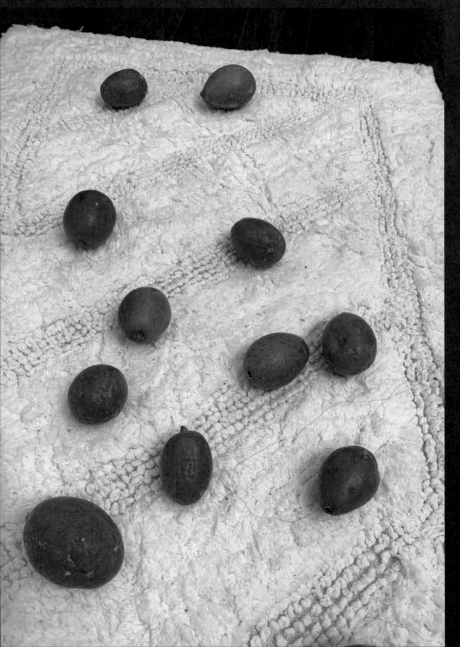

Y

YELLOW
SQUASH

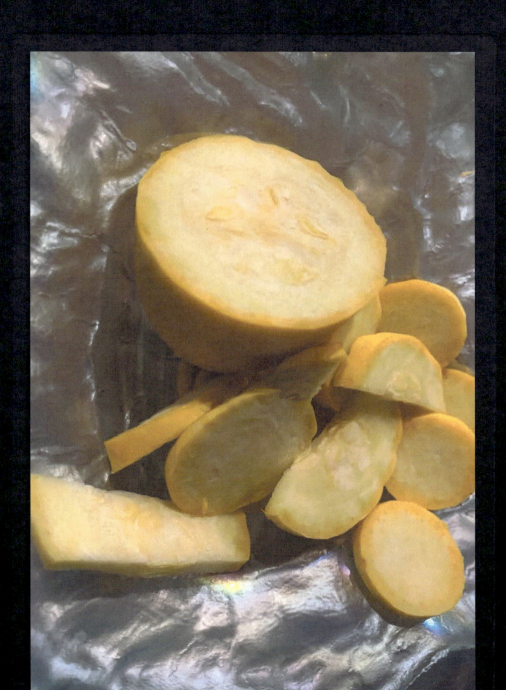

Z

ZUCCHINI

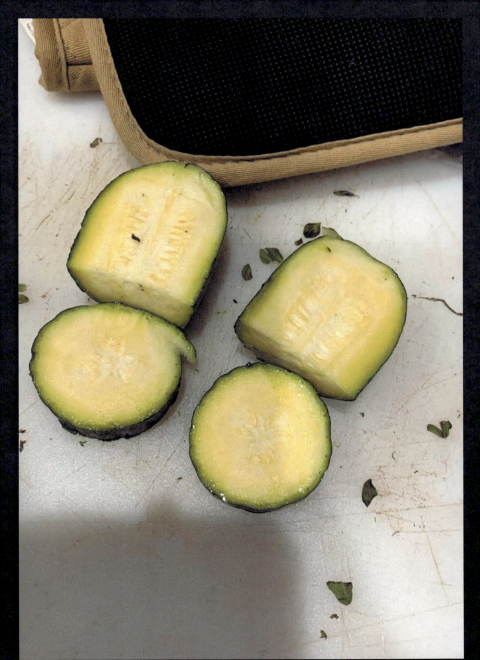

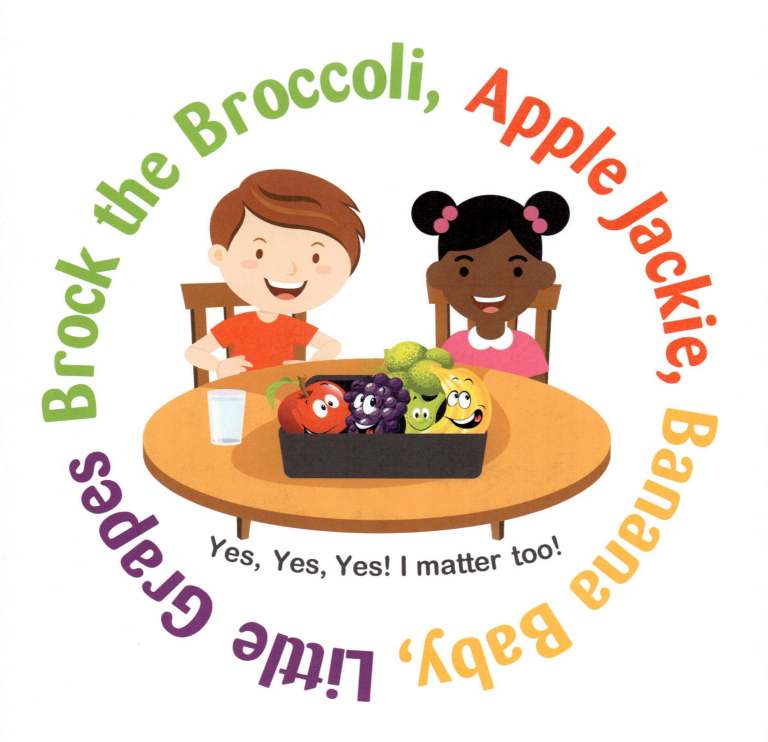

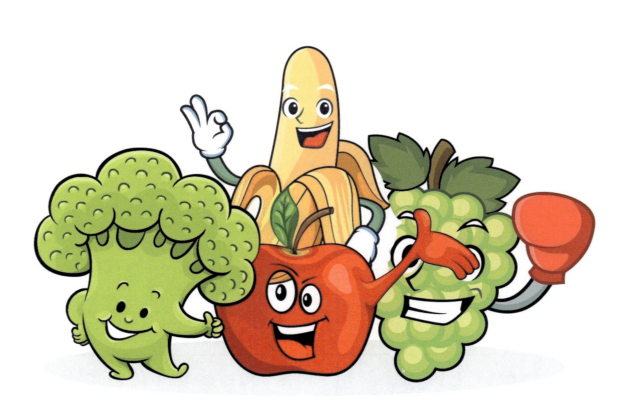

Fruits and Vegetables of the Alphabet

Asparagus	*Veggie*	Good for digestion
Broccoli	*Veggie*	Good for skin
Carrot	*Veggie*	Good for eyes
Dill	*Leaf*	Fights infection
Eggplant	*Veggie*	Good for your heart
Fig	*Fruit*	Good for bones
Grape	*Fruit*	Fight cancer cells
Honeydew	*Fruit*	Low in salt
Iceberg Lettuce	*Veggie*	Good for eyes
Jalapeno	*Fruit*	Repairs cells in the body
Kale	*Veggie*	Helps you grow and learn
Leek	*Veggie*	Helps you grow and learn
Mango	*Fruit*	Helps when you are sick

Napa Cabbage	*Veggie*	Helps when you are sick
Orange	*Fruit*	Fights cold and flu
Pea	*Veggie*	Good for skin and heart
Quinoa	*Fruit*	Helps bone and teeth
Rutabaga	*Veggie*	Prevents disease
Spinach	*Veggie*	Good for heart and brain
Tomato	*Fruit*	Fight disease
Ugli	*Fruit*	Keeps you healthy
Vanilla Bean	*Leaf*	Prevents gas
Watermelon	*Fruit*	Good for hydration
Ximenia	*Fruit*	Good for soft skin
Yellow Squash	*Fruit*	Good for headaches
Zucchini	*Fruit*	Helps your heart and stomach

A, B, C, D, E, F, G....

Do you know your fruits and veggies?

Name: _____

Draw a picture of your favorite fruit or veggie.